THE HIDDEN SIDE OF DIABETES

Natural ways to stop and reverse type 2 diabetes

BY

DR.MARY I. VERA

DISCLAIMER

TABLE OF CONTENTS

INTRODUCTION

Understanding Type 2 Diabetes

Type 2 diabetes is a chronic metabolic disorder characterized by elevated blood sugar levels due to insulin resistance and impaired insulin production. Its global prevalence is on the rise, primarily due to factors such as changing lifestyles, urbanization, and an aging population. The key distinction from Type 1 diabetes is that individuals with Type 2 diabetes often produce insulin but cannot use it effectively. Diabetes is an infection that happens when your blood glucose, likewise called glucose, is excessively high. Blood glucose is your principal wellspring of energy and comes from the food you eat. Insulin, a chemical made by the pancreas, assists glucose from food with getting into your cells to be utilized for energy.

Diabetes mellitus is described by strangely elevated degrees of sugar (glucose) in the blood.

At the point when how much glucose in the blood increments, e.g., after a feast, it sets off the arrival of the chemical insulin from the pancreas. Insulin animates muscle and fat cells to eliminate glucose from the blood and invigorates the liver to use glucose, causing the glucose level to diminish to typical levels.

In individuals with diabetes, glucose levels stay high. This might be on the grounds that insulin isn't being created by any means, isn't made at adequate levels, or isn't as powerful as it ought to be. The most widely recognized types of diabetes are type 1 diabetes (5%), which is an immune system problem, and type 2 diabetes (95%), which is related to corpulence. Gestational diabetes is a type of diabetes that happens in pregnancy.

Type 1 Diabetes

Additionally called insulin-subordinate diabetes mellitus (IDDM) or adolescent beginning diabetes.

Results when the body's safe framework assaults and obliterates its own insulin-creating beta cells in the pancreas.

Individuals with type 1 diabetes need a day-to-day infusion of insulin to live.

Grows most frequently in kids or youthful grown-ups.
In spite of the fact that hazard factors are not clear-cut, the immune system, hereditary, and ecological variables are associated with the illness' turn of events.

Type 2 Diabetes
Additionally called noninsulin-subordinate diabetes mellitus (NIDDM) or grown-up beginning diabetes.
Happens when the body makes sufficient insulin yet can't utilize it successfully.
Typically creates in grown-ups beyond 40 years old.

Around 90-95 percent of individuals with diabetes have type 2; around 80 percent are overweight.

More normal among more established; hefty individuals who have a family background of diabetes; have had gestational diabetes; and are of African American, Hispanic American, Asian American, Pacific Islander, and Local American nationalities.

Gestational Diabetes

Creates or is found during pregnancy. Normally vanishes when the pregnancy is finished.

Ladies who have had gestational diabetes have a more serious gamble of creating type 2 diabetes further down the roads

CHAPTER 1

Diabetes is connected with high glucose, yet various types of the problem have contrasting roots.

Type 1 Diabetes: An Autoimmune Origin

Type 1 diabetes, often referred to as juvenile-onset diabetes, typically develops in childhood or adolescence. This form of diabetes has an autoimmune origin. It occurs when the immune system mistakenly targets and destroys the insulin-producing beta cells in the pancreas. As a result, the body becomes deficient in insulin, and individuals with Type 1 diabetes rely on external insulin injections or pumps to regulate their blood sugar levels.

The precise trigger for this autoimmune response is not fully understood, but it is believed to involve a combination of genetic predisposition and environmental factors. Infections or exposure to certain viruses may play a role in initiating this autoimmune reaction. Type 1 diabetes is not preventable and currently has no cure; it necessitates lifelong insulin therapy.

Type 2 Diabetes: A Complex Interplay of Factors

In contrast, Type 2 diabetes is the more common form of diabetes, typically occurring in adulthood. It has a multifactorial origin, involving a complex interplay of genetic and lifestyle factors. While genetics plays a role in determining an individual's susceptibility to Type 2 diabetes, it is often exacerbated or triggered by poor lifestyle choices.

Obesity, physical inactivity, and an unhealthy diet are significant contributors to the development of Type 2 diabetes. Excess body fat, particularly around the abdomen, leads to insulin resistance, where the body's cells do not respond effectively to insulin. As a result, blood sugar levels rise, and the pancreas may eventually struggle to produce enough insulin to compensate.

Prevention and management of Type 2 diabetes primarily revolve around lifestyle modifications. This includes maintaining a healthy weight, engaging in regular physical activity, and making dietary choices that promote blood sugar control. In some cases, oral medications or insulin therapy may be prescribed to help manage the condition.

Diabetes, characterized by high glucose levels, has diverse origins depending on the type. Type 1 diabetes stems from an autoimmune response that destroys insulin-producing cells, while Type 2 diabetes is a result of genetic susceptibility exacerbated by poor lifestyle choices. Recognizing these differences is vital for early diagnosis, tailored treatment, and effective prevention strategies. Ultimately, whether Type 1 or Type 2, managing diabetes requires a comprehensive approach that encompasses medical care, lifestyle adjustments, and ongoing support.

CHAPTER 2

Like stoutness, type 2 diabetes can't be treated by basically restricting calorie admission.

Stoutness and type 2 diabetes cannot be effectively treated by simply restricting calorie intake. While calorie control is a crucial aspect of managing these conditions, the root causes often involve complex factors like insulin resistance, genetics, and hormonal imbalances. Successful treatment typically requires a multifaceted approach, including a balanced diet, regular physical activity, and in some cases, medication or insulin therapy to manage blood sugar levels. Lifestyle changes and addressing the underlying metabolic issues are key components of effective management. Furthermore, the idea that a one-size-fits-all approach of solely cutting calories may not address the specific needs of individuals with obesity and type 2 diabetes. Restricting calories alone can lead to muscle loss and nutritional deficiencies, which may exacerbate the underlying health problems.

A more holistic approach to treatment involves:

Diet Modification: Emphasizing a balanced diet that includes whole grains, lean proteins, fruits, vegetables, and healthy fats. Reducing sugar and processed foods is essential to control blood sugar levels.

Regular Exercise: Physical activity is crucial for improving insulin sensitivity and overall health. A combination of aerobic exercise and strength training can be particularly beneficial.

Weight Management: While weight loss can be a part of the strategy, it should be achieved gradually and in a sustainable way. Crash diets or extreme calorie restrictions can be harmful.

Medication: In some cases, medication or insulin therapy may be necessary to help control blood sugar levels. These should be prescribed and monitored by healthcare professionals.

Monitoring and Education: Regular monitoring of blood sugar levels, education on nutrition, and support from healthcare providers are essential for long-term success.

Individualized Approach: Recognizing that each person's needs and responses to treatment may vary, a personalized plan is crucial to address the unique challenges of obesity and type 2 diabetes.

Managing obesity and type 2 diabetes goes beyond calorie restriction. A comprehensive approach that considers lifestyle changes, dietary modifications, physical activity, and medical intervention when necessary is essential for effective treatment and improved health outcomes.

CHAPTER 3

Rising fructose utilization is a supporter of broad greasy liver infection.

The increasing consumption of fructose is indeed a contributing factor to the widespread occurrence of fatty liver disease. Fructose is a type of sugar found naturally in fruits and honey, but it is also a common component of high-fructose corn syrup (HFCS), which is used in many processed foods and sugary beverages.

Here's why rising fructose consumption is linked to fatty liver disease:

Metabolism: Unlike glucose, which is metabolized throughout the body, fructose is primarily processed by the

liver. Excessive fructose intake can overwhelm the liver's capacity to metabolize it, leading to the conversion of fructose into fat within the liver.
Fat Accumulation: The excessive fructose-derived fat is stored in the liver, resulting in the accumulation of triglycerides. This accumulation is a key driver of non-alcoholic fatty liver disease (NAFLD).
Insulin Resistance: High fructose consumption can lead to insulin resistance, which impairs the body's ability to regulate blood sugar and can further exacerbate fatty liver disease.
Inflammation: Fatty liver can trigger inflammation, which is associated with liver damage and can progress to more severe conditions like non-alcoholic steatohepatitis (NASH).

Obesity: Fructose consumption has
been linked to weight gain and obesity,
which are also risk factors for fatty liver
disease.

Reducing the consumption of foods and
beverages high in added sugars,
particularly those containing
high-fructose corn syrup, is an
important step in preventing and
managing fatty liver disease. A diet
focused on whole foods, including fruits
in their natural form, vegetables, and
lean proteins, can help reduce the risk
of fatty liver disease and its associated
health complications. Additionally,
lifestyle changes, such as regular
exercise and weight management, can
be beneficial in improving liver health.

CHAPTER 4

Insulin shots aren't the response to type 2 diabetes, on the grounds that an excessive amount of insulin is terrible for the body.

Insulin shots are not always the primary solution for managing type 2 diabetes, as the idea that "more insulin is better" is a misconception. While insulin therapy can be a crucial treatment for some individuals with type 2 diabetes, it's important to understand the nuances involved.

Here are some key points to consider:

Insulin Resistance: Many people with type 2 diabetes have insulin resistance, where their cells don't respond effectively to insulin. In these cases, providing more insulin through shots may not resolve the underlying problem.

Medication Options: Before resorting to insulin, healthcare providers often explore other options such as oral medications, injectable non-insulin medications, and lifestyle changes like diet and exercise. These treatments aim to improve blood sugar control without immediately relying on insulin.

Timing: The use of insulin can vary. It may be prescribed when other treatments have proven ineffective, or in cases where a person's blood sugar levels are dangerously high.

Balance: Excessive insulin can lead to hypoglycemia (low blood sugar), which can be dangerous. A careful balance is required to avoid both hyperglycemia (high blood sugar) and hypoglycemia.

Lifestyle Management: Lifestyle modifications, including diet and physical activity, are key components in managing type 2 diabetes. These changes can reduce the need for insulin or other medications.

Individualized Treatment: The approach to managing type 2 diabetes should be personalized, taking into account the individual's specific needs, health status, and response to different treatments.

Insulin shots are an important tool in managing type 2 diabetes, but they are not a one-size-fits-all solution, and they are not necessarily indicative of "too much insulin being better." The treatment approach should be based on the patient's unique circumstances and may include a combination of therapies, including lifestyle changes and other medications, to achieve optimal blood sugar control while minimizing potential risks. Consulting with a healthcare professional is essential to determine the most suitable treatment plan for each person with type 2 diabetes.

CHAPTER 5

Bariatric medical procedure can be a compelling remedy for type 2 diabetes, however it's not the most ideal arrangement by and large.

Bariatric surgery can indeed be an effective treatment for type 2 diabetes, especially in cases of severe obesity. However, it's important to recognize that it's not always the ideal solution for everyone, and it comes with both benefits and potential risks.

Here are some key points to consider:

Effectiveness: Bariatric surgery, such as gastric bypass or sleeve gastrectomy, can lead to rapid and significant weight loss, which often results in improved blood sugar control. Many individuals with type 2 diabetes see a remission of their diabetes symptoms after surgery.

Patient Selection: Bariatric surgery is typically recommended for individuals with a high body mass index (BMI) or those who have not responded well to other treatments. It is not a first-line treatment for type 2 diabetes in individuals with mild or moderate obesity.

Risks and Complications: Like any surgical procedure, bariatric surgery carries potential risks and complications. These can include infection, nutritional deficiencies, and the need for further surgeries.

Lifestyle Changes: Bariatric surgery is not a stand-alone solution. Patients must commit to significant lifestyle changes, including dietary modifications and regular physical activity, to maintain the benefits of the surgery and overall health.

Long-Term Outcomes: The long-term success of bariatric surgery in maintaining weight loss and diabetes remission can vary from person to person. It's not a guarantee of permanent results.

Consultation with Healthcare Professionals: Decisions about bariatric surgery should be made in consultation with healthcare providers, who can assess an individual's specific needs and circumstances.

bariatric surgery can be a powerful tool for managing type 2 diabetes in specific cases, especially when obesity is a significant factor. However, it's not the most appropriate solution for everyone, and it should be considered as part of a comprehensive treatment plan that includes lifestyle changes and regular medical monitoring. The decision to undergo bariatric surgery should be well-informed and made in close consultation with healthcare professionals.

CHAPTER 6

Anyway, how might you invert and forestall it? There are two exceptionally successful procedures you can take on today.

Certainly, reversing and preventing type 2 diabetes often involves making significant lifestyle changes. Here are two highly effective strategies you can start implementing today:

Healthy Eating:

Balanced Diet: Focus on a well-balanced diet that includes a variety of foods. Choose complex carbohydrates like whole grains, lean protein sources, plenty of vegetables, and fruits in moderation. Avoid or limit foods high in added sugars, saturated and trans fats.

Portion Control: Be mindful of portion sizes to avoid overeating. Smaller, regular meals can help stabilize blood sugar levels.

Carbohydrate Management: Monitor and control carbohydrate intake. Pay attention to the glycemic index of foods, which indicates how quickly they raise blood sugar.

Regular Physical Activity:

Exercise Routine: Incorporate regular physical activity into your daily life. Aim for at least 150 minutes of moderate-intensity aerobic exercise per week, such as brisk walking, swimming, or cycling.

Strength Training: Include strength or resistance training exercises at least two days a week. Building muscle can improve insulin sensitivity and help control blood sugar levels.

Consistency: Make exercise a consistent part of your routine to achieve lasting benefits.

Additionally, here are some important tips:

Weight Management: If overweight, losing excess weight can significantly improve insulin sensitivity and blood sugar control.

Monitor Blood Sugar: Regularly check your blood sugar levels as advised by your healthcare provider to track your progress and make necessary adjustments.

Medication: If prescribed by your healthcare provider, take medications as directed.

Stress Management: Stress can impact blood sugar levels. Practice stress-reduction techniques like mindfulness, meditation, or yoga.

Consult Healthcare Provider: Always consult with your healthcare provider or a registered dietitian for personalized guidance and to determine the best approach for your specific situation.

Reversing and preventing type 2 diabetes is possible, but it requires commitment and a long-term approach. These strategies can be highly effective, but it's essential to consult with healthcare professionals to create a tailored plan that suits your individual needs and to monitor your progress along the way.

CHAPTER 7

So what precisely does fasting include?

One chance is day to day segment control, yet that is presumably not the most fitting response. Restoring diabetes and empowering weight reduction aren't simple things to accomplish.

Consider an English report did in 2015: it examined the viability of typical nourishing guiding that zeroed in on segment control and presumed that this approach fizzled for 99.5 percent, everything being equal. They simply didn't lose a lot of weight.

The explanation it doesn't work is that bringing down day to day calorie consumption just dials back your metabolic rate while expanding your vibe of yearning. That is hard to persevere and eventually most health food nuts collapse and are rapidly back to their unique weight.

A vastly improved approach is irregular fasting.That is fundamentally about going without all food sources briefly, and could be anything from a day to seven days. From that point onward, individuals can get back to their ordinary weight control plans.

The work expected to follow this sort of plan is substantially more focused, which makes it simpler to carry out than the everyday routine of piece control. What's more, above all, it works!

Fasting causes a plunge in the body's insulin creation, meaning it stays insulin-delicate as opposed to fostering a protection from the chemical.

One more English review directed in 2011 by N.M. Harvie highlights the adequacy of this methodology. Harvie analyzed two gatherings of calorie counters. The primary ate a Mediterranean eating routine with a confined calorie consumption, while the second ate typically for five days every week and abstained for the other two. The two gatherings encountered some weight reduction following a half year, however the subsequent gathering likewise had a lot of lower insulin levels than the first.

This recommends that irregular fasting may be the best remedy for type 2 diabetes. All things considered, it's high insulin levels and insulin obstruction

which are liable for the problem and
fasting diminishes these.

Conclusion

Type 2 diabetes contrasts essentially from type 1 diabetes. While the last option is portrayed by low insulin levels, the previous is a result of hazardously high insulin levels which, thusly, prompts insulin opposition and a scope of serious medical problems. Fortunately type 2 diabetes can be switched. Consolidate carb evasion and an adjustment of diet with irregular fasting and you'll be well headed to recuperation.

Fasting is compelling, yet you want to track down a routine that works for you. Irregular fasting is an incredible approach to bringing down your insulin levels, however it takes a touch of tweaking to hit the nail on the head. In the event that you're new to the thought, begin by counseling a clinical or dietary master. The subsequent stage is to track down a routine that suits your digestion. Certain individuals like to quick for longer periods less every now and again, while others find more successive however more limited diets more viable. The key is testing. Take a stab at fasting for 3-4 days like clockwork, or just skipping supper and fasting for eighteen hours before breakfast. Furthermore, make sure to keep yourself very much hydrated during anything routine you go with and stop assuming you feel debilitated!